Ultimate Guide To The Mediterranean Diet

The Ultimate Guide To Discover The Easiest Way To Make Tasty Recipes For Weight Loss And Burning Fat

Written By

HOLLIE MCCARTHY, RDN

Table of Contents

INTRODUCTION

Thank you for purchasing this book!

Most of the studies done on the Mediterranean diet **have shown its effectiveness** in maintaining good general health. It has been widely demonstrated how the Mediterranean diet reduces the incidence of:

- colon cancer
- breast neoplasia
- diabetes
- infarction
- atherosclerosis
- hypertension
- digestive diseases
- inhibits metabolic syndrome - which is one of the main causes of the occurrence of cardiovascular diseases.

Enjoy your reading!

BREAKFAST

Maple sausage pancake muffins

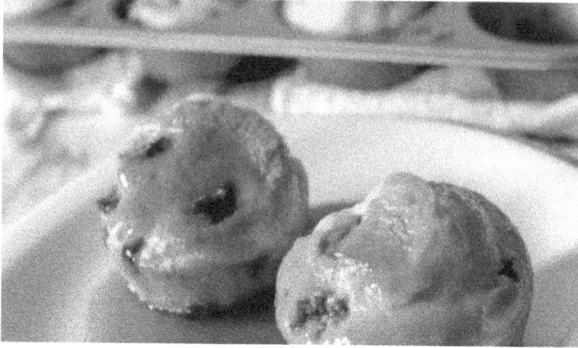

SERVES: 4

INGREDIENTS

- 6 oz. Ground Sausage
- 1 1/2 cups Honeyville Almond Flour
- 4 large Eggs
- 4 tbsp. Coconut Milk
- 4 tbsp. Maple Syrup
- 2 tbsp. Psyllium Husk Powder
- 1 tsp. Vanilla Extract
- 1 tsp. Baking Powder
- 1/4 tsp. Salt
- 20 drops Liquid Stevia
- 1/4 cup Erythritol
-

DIRECTIONS

1. If you happen to have some Jimmy Dean sausage, you can just cut the log in half and go ahead and start. If not, measure out 6 oz. Sausage and break it up into small pieces.
2. Turn a pan up to high heat and fry the outsides of the sausage until crisp.
3. You don't want the inside completely cooked since it will happen in the baking process.
4. Preheat your oven to 350F. Measure out 4 eggs, 4 tbsp. coconut milk, 4 tbsp. maple syrup, 1 tsp. vanilla extract and 20 drops of liquid stevia.
5. Mix this well, you want to make sure that all of the ingredients are well distributed.
6. Measure out the dry ingredients: 1 1/2 cup Honeyville Almond Flour, 1 tsp.
7. Baking Powder, 1/4 cup Erythritol, and 2 tbsp. Psyllium Husk powder.
8. Mix the wet and dry ingredients, and then mix all of the seared sausage pieces into the mixture.
9. Measure out the batter into 12 silicone cupcake molds. Put them into the oven and bake for 20-25 minutes.
10. Once cooked, remove from the oven and let cool for 5 minutes.
11. Remove from the silicone cupcake molds and let cool longer on a cooling rack (if you plan on storing in the fridge) or eat warm!
12. Add a drizzle of extra maple syrup if you'd like. Serve up!

NUTRITIONAL VALUES

160 Calories, 13g Fats, 1g Net Carbs, and 8g Protein.

Low carb blackberry pudding

SERVES: 2

INGREDIENTS

- 1/4 cup Coconut Flour
- 1/4 tsp. Baking Powder
- 5 large Egg Yolks
- 2 tbsp. Coconut Oil
- 2 tbsp. Butter
- 2 tbsp. Heavy Cream
- 2 tsp. Lemon Juice
- Zest 1 Lemon
- 1/4 cup Blackberries
- 2 tbsp. Erythritol
- 10 drops Liquid Stevia

DIRECTIONS

1. Preheat oven to 350F. Then, separate the egg yolks from the whites and set them aside. You can save the egg whites to make different things like Low Carb Coconut Shrimp!
2. Measure out 1/4 cup Coconut Flour, and 1/4 tsp. Baking Powder. Set aside.
3. Measure out 2 tbsp. Coconut Oil and 2 tbsp. Butter. Set aside.

4. Beat the egg yolks until they're pale in color. Then, add 2 tbsp. erythritol and 10 drops of liquid stevia. Beat again until fully combined.

5. Add 2 tbsp. heavy cream, 2 tsp. lemon juice, and the zest of 1 lemon.

6. Add the coconut and butter you had previously measured out and beat everything together until no lumps are found.

7. Sift the dry ingredients over the wet ingredients, then mix well at a slow speed.

8. Measure out the batter into 2 ramekins and lightly smash the blackberries with your finger. Distribute the blackberries evenly in the batter by pushing them into the top of the batter.

9. Bake for 20-25 minutes at 350F. Once finished, let cool for 5 minutes or so.

10. Pour some heavy whipping cream over the top and eat! It's super delicious on its own too! You can share the ramekin with another, or eat it by yourself.

NUTRITIONAL VALUES

475 Calories, 45g Fats, 5g Net Carbs,a nd 9g Protein.

Spinach, onion, and goat cheese omelette

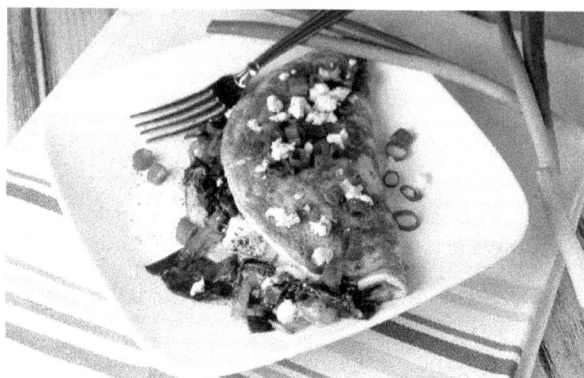

SERVES: 1

INGREDIENTS

- 1/4 medium Onion
- 2 tbsp. Butter
- 1 large handful of Spinach
- 3 large Eggs
- 2 tbsp. Heavy Cream
- 1 oz. Goat Cheese
- 1 medium Spring Onion (Garnish)
- Salt and pepper to Taste

DIRECTIONS

1. Spread out 2 tbsp. butter into a hot pan using your hands.

2. Cut 1/4 onion while the butter begins to brown. Slice into long strips.

3. Once the butter begins to brown, add onion to the pan and allow the onion to caramelize.

4. Once the onion is translucent, add 1 large handful of spinach (~2 cups) to the pan. Let this cook down and wilt. Season with salt and pepper to taste.

5. Remove the spinach and onion mixture from the pan and set aside. In a small measuring container, crack 3 large eggs.

6. Add 2 tbsp. heavy cream, salt, and pepper to the eggs. Mix this well.

7. Heat the pan to medium-low heat (it should already be hot). Add your egg mixture to the pan and allow it to cook.

8. Once the edges begin to set, add the onion and spinach mixture back into half of the omelet. Crumble 1 oz. goat cheese over the top of the spinach and season with more salt and pepper if you'd like.

9. Fold the omelet in half once the top begins to set and serve! Garnish with spring onions if you'd like.

NUTRITIONAL VALUES

620 Calories, 56g Fats, 5g Net Carbs, and 25g Protein.

Coconut cream yogurt

SERVES: 4

INGREDIENTS

- 1 can Full Fat Coconut Milk
- 2 capsules NOW Probiotic-ic-10
- 1/2 tsp. NOW Xanthan Gum (1/4 tsp. split between both jars)
- 2/3 cup Heavy Whipping Cream
- Toppings of Your Choice

DIRECTIONS

1. Open a can of coconut milk and stir it well. You want to make sure the cream and water in the can is thoroughly mixed.
2. Put the coconut milk into whatever container you'd like. I separated mine into 2 200mL mason jars. Have your NOW Probiotic-10 handy.
3. Break the capsules into the coconut milk. If you are using 2 jars, use 1 capsule per jar. If you are using 1 jar, use 2 capsules. Stir the mixture together well and place the lids on the jar.
4. Turn your oven light on and place the jars in the oven. Close the oven door, keeping the light on, and let it sit for 12-24 hours overnight. The longer the bacteria can culture, the thicker the mixture will get, but it doesn't make too big of a difference.
5. Empty your entire yogurt into a mixing bowl and sprinkle 1/2 tsp. Xanthan gum over it. Using a hand mixer, mix this well.

6. In a separate bowl, whip up 2/3 cup heavy cream until stiff peaks form. You want this to be solid cream almost.

7. Dump the solid cream into the yogurt and mix at a low speed until the consistency you want is achieved.

8. Add toppings, flavorings, or fillings of your choice, and enjoy!

9. Usually, yogurt has a serving size of 1/2 cup, but you will get just over 1/2 cup per serving with this.

NUTRITIONAL VALUES

315 Calories, 33g Fats, 3g Net Carbs and 0g Protein.

LUNCH

Crockpot Buffalo Chicken Soup

SERVES: 5

INGREDIENTS

- 3 medium Chicken Thighs, deboned and sliced (~2 lbs without bones)
- 1 tsp. Onion Powder
- 1 tsp. Garlic Powder
- 1/2 tsp. Celery Seed
- 1/4 cup butter
- 1/3 – 1/2 cup Frank's Hot Sauce (depending on how spicy you like it)
- 3 cups Beef Broth
- 1 cup Heavy Cream
- 2 oz. Cream Cheese
- 1/4 tsp. Xanthan Gum
- Salt and Pepper to Taste

DIRECTIONS

1. De-bone the chicken thighs
2. Cut or slice the chicken into chunks and drop them in the crockpot.
3. Add all the rest of the ingredients to the crockpot except for cream, cheese, and xanthan gum. Set crockpot on low for 6 hours (or high for 3 hours) and let cook completely.
4. Once everything is cooked, remove the chicken from the crockpot and shred using a fork.

5. Add cream, cheese, and xanthan gum to the crockpot. Using an immersion blender, emulsify all of the liquids together. This will help the soup from separating while you are eating.

6. Place the chicken back into the crockpot and stir together. Taste and season with extra salt, pepper, and hot sauce if you'd like.

7. Serve up and enjoy!

NUTRITIONAL VALUES

523 Calories, 42g Fats, 4g Net Carbs, and 20.8g Protein.

Roasted red bell pepper and cauliflower soup

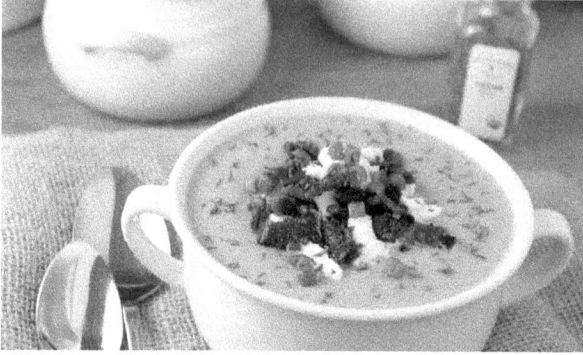

SERVES: 5

INGREDIENTS

- 2 medium Red Bell Peppers, cut in half and de-seeded
- 1/2 head Cauliflower, cut into florets
- 2 tbsp. Duck Fat
- 3 medium Green Onions, diced
- 3 cups Chicken Broth
- 1/2 cup Heavy Cream
- 4 tbsp. Duck Fat
- 1 tsp. Garlic Powder
- 1 tsp. Dried Thyme
- 1 tsp. Smoked Paprika
- 1/4 tsp. Red Pepper Flakes
- 4 oz. Goat Cheese, crumbled (to top)

- Salt and Pepper to Taste

DIRECTIONS

1. Put the oven on the broil setting. Slice peppers in half and de-seed them. Lay them skin side up on a foil-covered baking tray and broil for 10-15 minutes or until the skin is charred and blackened.
2. While peppers are broiling, cut cauliflower into florets. If the florets are large, cut florets in half or quarters.
3. Once peppers are done, remove them from the oven and place them in a container with a lid, or a food saver bag, and seal. Let the peppers steam and cook longer to soften while cauliflower roasts.
4. Use 2 tbsp. melted duck fat, salt, and pepper to season the cauliflower. Roast cauliflower in 400F oven for 30-35 minutes.
5. Remove the skins from the peppers by peeling them off carefully.
6. In a pot, bring 4 tbsp. duck fat to heat and add diced green onion. Once the green onion is slightly cooked, add seasonings into the pan to toast.
7. Add chicken broth, red pepper, and cauliflower to the pan. Let this simmer for 10-20 minutes.
8. Take an immersion blender to the mixture. Make sure that all fats are emulsified with the   mixture by the time you're finished – about 1-2 minutes.
9. Season to taste, and then add cream and mix.
10. Serve with some crispy bacon and goat's cheese. Garnish with extra thyme and green onion.

NUTRITIONAL VALUES.

345 Calories, 32g Fats, 2g Net Carbs, and 4g Protein.

DINNER

Chicken pad thai

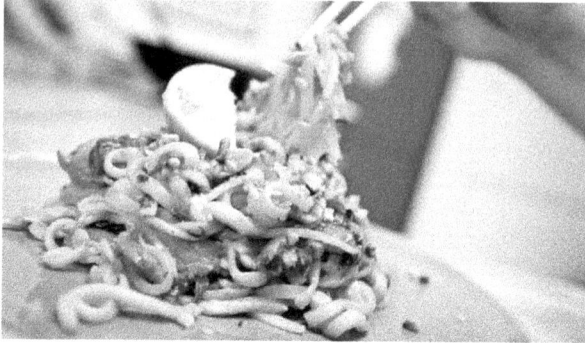

SERVES: 4

INGREDIENTS

Pad Thai Sauce

- Juice 1/2 Lime
- Juice 1/3 Lemon
- 1/2 tbsp. Reduced Sugar
- 1/2 tsp. Worcestershire

Sauce

- 3 tbsp. Red Boat Fish Sauce
- 1/2 tbsp. Sambal Olek
- 1/2 tsp. Minced Garlic
- 1 tbsp. Natural Peanut Butter
- 1 tsp. Rice Wine Vinegar
- 7 drops Liquid Stevia

Noodles and Toppings

- 1/4 cup Cilantro, chopped

- 3 medium Green Onions, chopped

- 2 large Eggs

- 2 packets Shirataki Noodles

- 3 medium Chicken Thighs

- 4 tbsp. Coconut Oil

- 4 oz. Mung Bean Sprouts

- 2 tbsp. Peanuts, chopped

DIRECTIONS

1   Mix all of the ingredients for the sauce using a fork or whisk. Set aside.

2   Drain shirataki noodles and rinse well with hot water. Do this about 5 or 6 times, and then dry as much as you can using a cloth.

3   To get out extra moisture from the noodles, wring them out using a kitchen towel. Wring them out as much as possible to get rid of the excess moisture.

4   Debone chicken thighs. Start by cutting a line in the chicken where the bone is using kitchen shears. Cut all of the meat away from the bone, and then remove it by the bone by cutting around each end.

5   Once the chicken thighs are deboned, remove the skin and cut into cubed pieces.

6   Heat 2 tbsp. Coconut Oil in a pan over medium-high heat. Once the pan is hot, add the chicken to create a sear. Make sure not to overcrowd the pan

7   Flip the chicken pieces over to create a sear on the other side. Remove chicken from the pan (including the oil), and repeat using more coconut oil. Set chicken aside in a bowl.

8   Chop green onion and cilantro so that you're ready to use it.

9   In the same pan, you used to cook the chicken, add the shirataki noodles and dry fry them for 5-8 minutes or until noodles become firmer to the touch.

10 Reduce the heat of the pan, and add 2 eggs that have been whisked into the pan. Mix so that the eggs become scrambled and broken apart.

NUTRITIONAL VALUES

431 Calories, 33g Fats, 5g Net Carbs, and 23g Protein.

Crispy sesame beef

SERVES: 4

INGREDIENTS

- 1 medium Daikon Radish
- 1 lb. Ribeye Steak, sliced into ¼" strips
- 1 tbsp. Coconut Flour
- 1/2 tsp. Guar Gum
- 1 tbsp. Coconut Oil
- 4 tbsp. Soy Sauce
- 1 tsp. Sesame Oil
- 1 tsp. Oyster Sauce
- 1 tbsp. + 1 tsp. Rice Vinegar
- 1 tsp. Sriracha or Sambal Olek and ½ tsp. Red Pepper Flakes
- 1 tbsp. Toasted Sesame Seeds
- ½ medium Red Pepper, sliced into thin strips
- ½ medium Jalapeno Pepper, sliced into thin rings
- 1 medium Green Onion, chopped
- 1 clove Garlic, minced
- 1 tsp. Ginger, minced
- 7 drops Liquid Stevia
- Oil for frying

DIRECTIONS

1   Begin by preparing the daikon noodles for this recipe. Using a spiralizer, slice the daikon radish so that you're left with noodle-like strings. Once you've peeled the entire daikon radish, soak the daikon noodles in a bowl of cold water for 20 minutes.

2   Chop rib-eye steak into small strips, about 1/4 in thickness.

3   Place the rib eye steak in a bowl and pour the coconut flour and guar gum over the meat to coat all the pieces. This flour will act as light bread rings, green onion into small pieces, and mince the garlic and ginger.

4   Prepare all vegetables. Slice Red Pepper into thin strips, jalapeno into thin rings

5   In a wok pan or large skillet, heat coconut oil over medium heat. Once hot, add garlic, ginger, and red pepper strips. Fry for 2 minutes until aromatic, taking care not to burn. Add the soy sauce, oyster sauce, sesame oil, rice vinegar, stevia, and sriracha. Whisk to combine and allow to cook down for 1-2 minutes. Then add sesame seeds and red pepper flakes to the sauce mixture and stir.

6   While vegetables are cooking, heat 1" of cooking oil in a large pot or fryer over high heat until it reaches 325 degrees F. Once the oil reaches the proper temperature, add beef strips, making sure not to crowd the pot. With this shallow fry technique, you will need to turn the meat in the pan once to allow both sides to cook evenly. Fry for 2-3 minutes on each side, or until the meat begins to develop a deep brown crust.

7   Remove the beef from the oil and place on paper towels to absorb some of the oil.

8   Next, drop the cooked crispy beef into the wok pan containing the sauce and stir to combine. Cook for an additional 2 minutes to develop the flavors of the meat and sauce together.

9   Drain the daikon radish noodles and divide them onto each serving plate.

10   Top each with a portion of the sesame beef. Garnish with jalapeno slices and green onion.

NUTRITIONAL VALUES

412 calories, 33g Fats, 5g Net Carbs, and 25g Protein.

SNACKS

Maple pecan fat bomb bars

SERVES: 12

INGREDIENTS

- 2 cups Pecan Halves
- 1 cup Almond Flour
- 1/2 cup Golden Flaxseed Meal
- 1/2 cup Unsweetened Shredded Coconut
- 1/2 cup Coconut Oil
- 1/4 cup "Maple Syrup"
- 1/4 tsp. Liquid Stevia (~25 drops)

DIRECTIONS

1. Measure out 2 cups of pecan halves and bake for 6-8 minutes at 350F in the oven. Just enough to when they start becoming aromatic.
2. Remove pecans from the oven, then add to a plastic bag. Use a rolling pin to crush them into chunks. It doesn't matter too much about the consistency,
3. Mix the dry ingredients into a bowl: 1 cup Almond Flour, 1/2 cup Golden Flaxseed Meal, and 1/2 cup Unsweetened Shredded Coconut.
4. Add the crushed pecans to the bowl and mix them again.
5. Finally, add the 1/2 cup Coconut Oil, 1/4 cup "Maple Syrup" and 1/4 tsp. Liquid Stevia. Mix this well until a crumbly dough is formed.
6. Press the dough into a casserole dish. I am using an 11×7 baking dish for this.
7. Bake for 20-25 minutes at 350F, or until the edges are lightly browned.

8. Remove from the oven, allow to partially cool, and refrigerate for at least 1 hour (to cut cleanly).

9. Cut into 12 slices and remove using a spatula.

NUTRITIONAL VALUES

303 Calories, 30.5g Fats, 2g Net Carbs, and 9g Protein.

Low carb chia seed crackers

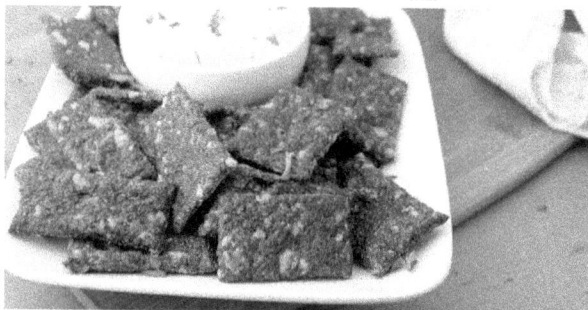

SERVES: 6

INGREDIENTS

- 1/2 cup Chia Seeds, ground
- 3 oz. Shredded Cheddar Cheese
- 1 1/4 cup Ice Water
- 2 tbsp. Psyllium Husk Powder
- 2 tbsp. Olive Oil
- 1/4 tsp. Xanthan Gum
- 1/4 tsp. Garlic Powder
- 1/4 tsp. Onion Powder
- 1/4 tsp. Oregano
- 1/4 tsp. Paprika
- 1/4 tsp. Salt
- 1/4 tsp. Pepper

DIRECTIONS

1. Preheat oven to 375F. Grind 1/2 cup Chia Seeds in a spice grinder. You want a meal like texture.

2. Add ground Chia Seeds, 2 tbsp. Psyllium Husk Powder, 1/4 tsp. Xanthan Gum, 1/4 tsp. Garlic Powder, 1/4 tsp. Onion Powder, 1/4 tsp. Oregano, 1/4 tsp. Paprika, 1/4 tsp. Salt and 1/4 tsp. Pepper to a bowl. Mix this together well.

3. Add 2 tbsp. Olive Oil to the dry ingredients and mix it together. It should turn into the consistency of wet sand.

4. Add 1 1/4 cup ice cold water to the bowl. Mix it together very well. You

5. may need to spend extra time mixing it together as the chia seeds and psyllium take a little bit of time to absorb the water. Keep mixing until a solid dough is formed.

6. Grate 3 oz. Cheddar Cheese and add it to the bowl.

7. Using your hands, knead the dough together. You want it to be relatively dry and not sticky by the time you finish.

8. Put the dough onto a silpat and let it sit for a few minutes.

9. Spread or roll the dough out thin so that it covers the entire silpat. If you can get it thinner, keep rolling and save the excess for a second cook.

10. Bake for 30-35 minutes in the oven until cooked.

11. Taken them out of the oven, and while hot, cut into individual crackers.

12. You can either use the blunt edge of a knife (don't cut into the silicone), or a large spatula.

13. Put the crackers back into the oven for 5-7 minutes on broil or until the tops are browned and well crisped. Remove from the oven and set on a rack to cool. As they cool, they get crisper.

14. Serve up with your favorite sauces. I'm using my Roasted Garlic Chipotle Aioli.

NUTRITIONAL VALUES

Per cracker, these are 31 calories, 5g Fats, 0.1g Net Carbs, and 3g Protein.

SIDE DISHES

Bacon wrapped asparagus with garlic aioli

SERVES: 1

INGREDIENTS

Bacon-Wrapped Asparagus

- 1 1/2 lb. Asparagus

- slices Bacon

- 2 tbsp. Olive Oil

- Kosher Salt

- Cracked Black Pepper

- Red Chili Flakes

Simple Garlic Aioli

- 2 tsp. Minced Garlic

- 1/4 tsp. Kosher Salt

- 1/4 cup Mayonnaise

- 1 large Egg Yolk

- 2 tsp. Fresh Lemon Juice

- Rendered Bacon Fat & Olive

- Oil

DIRECTIONS

1   Preheat the oven to 400F. Get the 1 1/2 lb. of asparagus out and prep it. If needed, cut off the bottom 1 inch of the stalks to allow for better consistency. The bottoms of asparagus are usually much thicker and harder than the rest of the stalk, meaning that it will be harder when it comes out of the oven.

2   My preference is to cut off this part of the stalk (normally a bit lighter in color).

3   Separate the asparagus into bundles. You should end up with 6 bundles with about 11 stalks per bundle. I was using small and thin stalks of asparagus.

4   If you're using larger asparagus, you may only get 4-5 stalks per bundle.

5   Wrap each bundle in 1 strip of bacon. Hold the tops of the spears of asparagus in your hand, then starting at the bottom wrap the asparagus in bacon. {

6   Move your way up until the whole slice of bacon wraps around the asparagus.

7   Transfer the now bacon wrapped asparagus on to a baking sheet wrapped in foil. Drizzle 2 tbsp. Olive Oil over the asparagus then seasons with salt, pepper, and red chili flakes.

8   Bake the asparagus at 400F for 20-22 minutes, then broil for an additional 2-5 minutes until the bacon is crisped and cooked.

9   Remove asparagus from the oven to let cool slightly.

10 Combine the rendered fats from the baking sheet, 2 tsp. minced garlic, 1 large egg yolk, and 2 tsp. fresh lemon juice in a small container.

11 Add the 1/4 cup mayonnaise and 1/4 tsp. salt, then mix until aioli is smooth.

12 Serve up and enjoy!

Cheesy bacon bombs

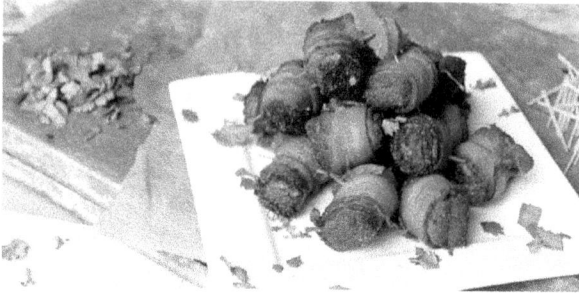

SERVES: 4

INGREDIENTS

- oz. Mozzarella Cheese
- tbsp. Almond Flour
- tbsp. Butter, melted
- 3 tbsp. Psyllium Husk Powder
- 1 large Egg
- 1/4 tsp. Salt
- 1/4 tsp. Fresh Ground Black pepper
- 1/8 tsp. Garlic Powder
- 1/8 tsp. Onion Powder
- slices Bacon
- 1 cup Oil, Lard, or Tallow(for frying)

DIRECTIONS

1. Add 4 oz. (half) Mozzarella cheese to a bowl.

2. Microwave 4 tbsp. butter for 15-20 seconds or until it is melted completely.

3. Microwave cheese for 45-60 seconds until melted and gooey (should be a

4. Add 1 egg and butter to the mixture and mix well.

5. Add 4 tbsp. almond flour, 3 tbsp. Psyllium husk, and the rest of your spices to the mixture (1/4 tsp. Salt, 1/4 tsp. Fresh Ground Black pepper, 1/8 tsp. Garlic Powder, and 1/8 tsp. Onion Powder).

6. Mix everything and dump it out onto a Silpat. Roll the dough out, or using your hands, form dough into a rectangle.

7. Spread the rest of the cheese over half of the dough and fold the dough over lengthwise.

8. Fold the dough again vertically so you form a square shape.

9. Crimp the edges using your fingers and press the dough together into a rectangle. You want the filling to be tight inside.

10. Using a knife, cut the dough into 20 squares.

11. Cut each slice of bacon in half, then lay the square at the end of 1 piece of bacon.

12. Roll the dough into the bacon tightly until the ends are overlapping. You can "stretch" your bacon if you need to before rolling.

13. Use a toothpick to secure the bacon after you roll it.

14. Do this for every piece of dough that you have. In the end, you will have 20 cheesy bacon bombs.

15. Heat oil, lard, or tallow to 350-375F, and then fry the cheesy bacon bombs 3 or 4 pieces at a time.

16. Remove to a paper towel to drain and cool once finished.

17   Serve up!

This makes a total of 20 Cheesy Bacon Bombs.

NUTRITIONAL VALUES

Each comes out to be 89 Calories, 2g Fats, 0.6g Net Carbs, and 5g Protein.

DESSERT

"Sour Cream" Coffee Cake

SERVES: 8

- ¾ cup chopped walnuts
- 1½ teaspoons ground cinnamon
- 2 cups sugar
- 2 cups all-purpose flour
- 2 teaspoons baking powder
- 1½ teaspoons baking soda
- Pinch salt
- 1 (12-ounce) package firm silken tofu, drained
- 2 teaspoons fresh lemon juice
- ½ cup canola or other neutral oil
- 1½ teaspoons pure vanilla extract
- ¾ cup vegan margarine

DIRECTIONS

1. Preheat the oven to 350°F. Grease a tube pan and set it aside. In a small bowl, combine the walnuts, cinnamon, and ¾ cup of the sugar and set aside.

2. In a medium bowl, sift together the flour, baking powder, baking soda, and salt and set aside.

3. In a food processor or blender, combine the tofu, lemon juice, canola oil, and vanilla, and blend until smooth.

4. In a large bowl, combine the margarine with the remaining 1¼ cups sugar and beat with an electric mixer on high until light and fluffy. Add the flour mixture and the tofu mixture and beat on low speed until blended. Increase the speed to medium, and beat for 3 more minutes.

5. Spread half of the batter in the prepared pan and sprinkle with half of the walnut mixture. Spread the remaining batter evenly over top and sprinkle with the remaining walnut mixture. Bake until firm and a toothpick inserted in the center comes out clean, approximately 60 minutes. If using a tube pan, let the cake cool in the pan for 10 minutes, before inverting the pan onto a wire rack to allow the cake to cool completely. If using a 9 x 13 pan, let the cake cool completely in the pan.

Hot Banana Ice Cream Cake

SERVES: 8

INGREDIENTS

- 1¼ cups broken vegan vanilla cookies
- ¾ cup pecan pieces
- ¼ cup plus 3 tablespoons vegan margarine
- 1-quart vegan vanilla ice cream softened
- ¼ cup light brown sugar
- 3 to 4 firm bananas, cut into ¼-inch slices
- ¼ cup dark rum or ¼ cup pineapple juice

DIRECTIONS

1. Grease the bottom and sides of a 9-inch springform pan and set it aside. In a food processor, combine the cookies and ¼ cup of the pecans and pulse until finely ground. Melt the ¼ cup of the margarine and add to the crumb mixture. Pulse to combine and moisten the crumbs. Press the crumb mixture into the bottom of the prepared pan and set aside.

2. Press the ice cream into the prepared crust, smoothing the top with a rubber spatula. Freeze for 3 hours to firm up.

3. Remove the cake from the freezer, remove the sides of the springform pan, and cut the cake into 8 slices. Fasten the sides back onto the pan and return the cake to the freezer until ready to serve.

4. Remove the sides of the springform pan and place the frozen cake slices on 8 dessert plates and set aside. In a medium skillet, combine the remaining 3 tablespoons margarine, remaining ½ cup

5. pecans, and sugar and cook over medium heat. Cook, stirring, until the sugar dissolves, about 1 minute. Add the banana slices and cook until slightly browned and softened but not mushy, about 1 minute. Carefully add the rum. Continue to cook the sauce until the alcohol mostly evaporates, 1 to minutes.

6. Spoon the bananas and sauce over each of the cake slices and serve immediately.

White Cupcakes With Variations

INGREDIENTS

- ¾ cup plain or vanilla soy milk
- 1½ teaspoons apple cider vinegar
- 1¼ cups all-purpose flour
- 1 teaspoon baking powder
- ¼ teaspoon baking soda
- ¼ teaspoon salt
- ¾ cup sugar
- ¼ cup canola or other neutral oil
- 1½ teaspoons pure vanilla extract

DIRECTIONS

1. Preheat the oven to 350°F. Line a 12-cup muffin tin with paper or foil cupcake liners. Set aside.

2. In a small bowl, combine the soy milk and vinegar and set aside. In a medium bowl, combine the flour, baking powder, baking soda, and salt. Mix to combine.

3. In a large bowl, combine the sugar, oil, and vanilla. Stir in the soy milk mixture. Add the dry ingredients to the wet ingredients and stir until smooth.

4. Pour the batter evenly into the prepared tin, about two-thirds full, and bake until a toothpick inserted in the center of a cupcake comes out clean, about 20 minutes. Cool completely before frosting.

This makes 12 cupcakes

Pumpkin Pie with a Hint Of Rum

SERVES: 8

INGREDIENTS

Crust

- 1¼ cups all-purpose flour
- ¼ teaspoon salt
- ½ teaspoon sugar
- ½ cup vegan margarine, cut into small pieces
- 3 tablespoons ice water, plus more if needed

Filling

- 1 (16-ounce) can solid pack pumpkin
- 1 (12-ounce) package extra-firm silken tofu, drained and patted dry
- 1 cup sugar
- Prepared egg replacement mixture for 2 eggs (see Vegan Baking)
- 1 tablespoon dark rum
- 1 tablespoon cornstarch
- 2 teaspoons ground cinnamon
- ½ teaspoon ground allspice
- ½ teaspoon ground ginger
- ½ teaspoon ground nutmeg

DIRECTIONS

1. In a medium bowl, combine the flour, salt, and sugar. Use a pastry blender or fork to cut in the margarine until the mixture resembles coarse crumbs. Add the water a little at a time and blend until the dough just starts to hold together. Flatten the dough into a round disk and wrap it in plastic wrap. Refrigerate for 30 minutes while you prepare the filling.

2. In a food processor, combine the pumpkin and tofu until well blended. Add the sugar, egg replacer, maple syrup, rum, cornstarch, cinnamon, allspice, ginger, and nutmeg, mixing until smooth and well combined.

3. Preheat the oven to 400°F. Roll out the dough on a lightly floured work surface to about 10 inches in diameter. Fit the dough into a 9-inch pie plate and trim and flute the edges.

4. Pour the filling into the crust. Bake for 15 minutes, then reduce the oven temperature to 350°F and bake for another 30 to 45 minutes, or until the filling is set. Let cool to room temperature on a wire rack, then chill in the refrigerator for 4 hours or longer.

Sweet Potato Pie

SERVES: 8

INGREDIENTS

Crust

- 1¼ cups all-purpose flour
- ¼ teaspoon salt
- ½ teaspoon sugar
- ½ cup vegan margarine, cut into small pieces
- 2 tablespoons ice water, or more if needed

Filling

- 2 cups mashed sweet potatoes
- 1 (12-ounce) package extra-firm silken tofu, drained and patted dry
- 1 cup light brown sugar
- Prepared egg replacement mixture for 2 eggs (see Vegan Baking)
- 1 tablespoon cornstarch
- 2 teaspoons ground cinnamon
- ½ teaspoon ground allspice
- ½ teaspoon ground ginger
- ½ teaspoon ground nutmeg

DIRECTIONS

1. Make the crust: In a large bowl, combine the flour, salt, and sugar. Use a pastry blender or fork to cut in the margarine until the mixture resembles coarse crumbs. Add the water a little at a time and blend until the dough just starts to hold together.

2. Flatten the dough into a disk and wrap it in plastic wrap. Refrigerate for 30 minutes while you prepare the filling.

3. Preheat the oven to 400°F.

4. Make the filling: In a food processor, combine the sweet potatoes and tofu until well blended. Add the sugar, egg replacer, maple syrup, cornstarch, cinnamon, allspice, ginger, and nutmeg, mixing until smooth and well combined.

5. Roll out dough on a lightly floured work surface to about 10 inches in diameter. Fit the dough into a 9-inch pie plate and trim and crimp the edges.

6. Pour the filling into the crust and bake for 15 minutes. Then turn to reduce the oven temperature to 350°F and bake for another 35 to 45 minutes, or until the filling is set.

Pecan Pie

SERVES: 8

INGREDIENTS

Crust

- 1¼ cups all-purpose flour
- ¼ teaspoon salt
- ½ teaspoon sugar
- ½ cup vegan margarine, cut into small pieces
- tablespoons ice water, plus more if needed

Filling

- 2 tablespoons cornstarch
- 1 cup water
- 1¼ cups pure maple syrup
- ½ teaspoon salt
- 2 tablespoons vegan margarine
- 1 teaspoon pure vanilla extract
- 2 cups unsalted pecan halves, toasted

DIRECTIONS

1. Make the crust: In a large bowl, combine the flour, salt, and sugar. Use a pastry blender or fork to cut in the margarine until the mixture resembles coarse crumbs. Add the water a little at a time and blend until the dough just starts to hold together.

2. Flatten the dough into a disk and wrap it in plastic wrap. Refrigerate for 30 minutes while you prepare the filling. Preheat the oven to 400°F.

3. Make the filling: In a small bowl, combine the cornstarch and the ¼ cup water and set aside. In a

4. medium saucepan, combine the remaining ¾ cup water and maple syrup, and bring to a boil over high heat. Boil for 5 minutes, then add the salt and the cornstarch mixture, whisking vigorously. Keep stirring and cook over high heat until the mixture thickens and becomes clear. Remove from the heat and stir in the margarine and vanilla.

5. Roll out the dough on a lightly floured work surface to about 10 inches in diameter. Fit the dough into a 9-inch pie plate. Trim the dough and flute the edges. Prick holes in the bottom of the dough with a fork. Bake until golden, about 10 minutes, then remove from the oven and set aside. Reduce the oven temperature to 350°F.

6. Once the margarine is melted, pour the filling into the prebaked crust. Arrange half the pecans in the filling, pressing them into the mixture and arranging the remaining half on the top of the pie. Bake for 30 minutes. Cool on a rack for about 1 hour, then refrigerate until chilled.

Peach Crumb Pie

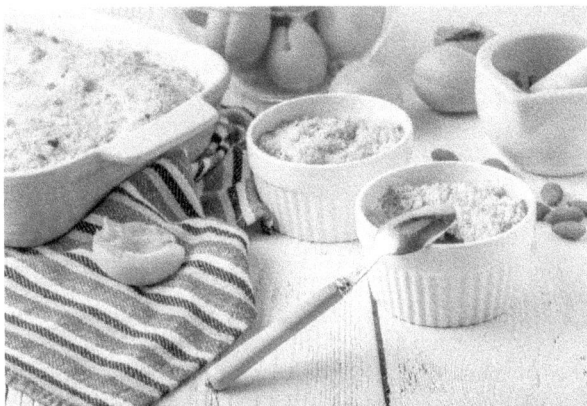

SERVES: 8

INGREDIENTS

- 1¼ cups all-purpose flour
- ¼ teaspoon salt
- ½ teaspoon sugar
- ½ cup vegan margarine, cut into small pieces
- 2 tablespoons cold water, plus more if needed
- ripe peaches, peeled, pitted, and sliced
- 1 teaspoon vegan margarine
- 2 tablespoons sugar
- ½ teaspoon ground cinnamon

DIRECTIONS

Topping

- ¾ cup old-fashioned oats
- ⅓ cup vegan margarine, softened
- 2 tablespoons sugar
- 1 teaspoon ground cinnamon
- ¼ teaspoon salt

DIRECTIONS

1. Make the crust: In a large bowl, combine the flour, salt, and sugar. Use a pastry blender or fork to cut in the margarine until the mixture resembles coarse crumbs. Add the water a little at a time and blend until the dough just starts to hold together.
2. Flatten the dough into a disk and wrap it in plastic wrap. Refrigerate for 30 minutes while you prepare the filling.
3. Preheat the oven to 425°F. Roll out the dough on a lightly floured work surface to about 10 inches in diameter. Fit the dough in a 9-inch pie plate and trim and crimp the edges. Arrange the peach slices in the crust. Dot with the margarine and sprinkle with sugar and cinnamon. Set aside.
4. Make the topping: In a medium bowl, combine the oats, margarine, sugar, cinnamon, and salt. Mix well and sprinkle on top of the fruit.
5. Bake until the fruit is bubbly and the crust is golden brown, about 40 minutes. Remove from oven and cool slightly 15 to 20 minutes. Serve warm.

White Chocolate Hazelnut Pie

SERVES: 8

INGREDIENTS

- 1½ cups vegan vanilla or chocolate cookie crumbs
- 1 cup vegan white chocolate chips or pieces, homemade (see Vegan White Chocolate) or store-bought
- ¼ cup water
- 2 tablespoons Frangelico (hazelnut liqueur)
- ounces extra-firm silken tofu, drained
- ¼ cup agave nectar
- 1 teaspoon pure vanilla extract
- ½ cup crushed toasted hazelnuts, for garnish
- ½ cup fresh berries, for garnish

DIRECTIONS

1 Grease an 8-inch pie plate or springform pan and set aside. In a food processor, combine the cookie crumbs and margarine and pulse until the crumbs are moistened. Press the crumb mixture into the bottom and sides of the prepared pan. Refrigerate until needed.

2 Melt the white chocolate in a double boiler over low heat, stirring constantly. Set aside.

3   In a high-speed blender, grind the cashews to a powder. Add the water and Frangelico and blend until smooth. Add the tofu, agave nectar, and vanilla and blend until smooth. Add the melted white chocolate and process until creamy.

4   Spread the mixture into the prepared pan. Cover and refrigerate for 3 hours, until well chilled. To serve, garnish with crushed hazelnuts and fresh berries.

Chocolate Mint Espresso Pie

SERVES: 8

INGREDIENTS

- 2 cups vegan chocolate cookies or mint-flavored chocolate sandwich cookies
- 1 (12-ounce) package vegan semisweet chocolate chips
- 1 (12.3-ounce) package firm silken tofu, drained and crumbled
- 2 tablespoons pure maple syrup or agave nectar
- 2 tablespoons plain or vanilla soy milk
- 2 tablespoons crème de menthe
- 2 teaspoons instant espresso powder

DIRECTIONS

1   Preheat the oven to 350°F. Lightly oil an 8-inch pie plate and set it aside.

2   If using sandwich cookies, carefully take them apart, reserving the cream filling in a separate bowl. Finely grind the cookies in a food processor. Add the vegan margarine and pulse until well incorporated.

3   Press the crumb mixture into the bottom of the prepared pan. Bake for 5 minutes. If using sandwich cookies, while the crust is still hot, spread the reserved cream filling over top of the crust. Set aside to cool, for 5 minutes.

4   Melt the chocolate chips in a double boiler or microwave. Set aside.

5   In a blender or food processor, combine the tofu, maple syrup, soy milk, crème de menthe, and espresso powder. Process until smooth.

6   Blend the melted chocolate into the tofu mixture until completely incorporated. Spread the filling into the prepared crust. Refrigerate for at least 3 hours to set before serving.

Strawberry Cloud Pie

SERVES: 8

INGREDIENTS

Crust

- 1¼ cups all-purpose flour
- ¼ teaspoon salt
- ½ teaspoon sugar
- ½ cup vegan margarine, cut into small pieces
- 3 tablespoons ice water

Filling

- 1 (12-ounce) package firm silken tofu, drained and pressed
- ¾ cup sugar
- 1 teaspoon pure vanilla extract
- 2 cups sliced fresh strawberries
- ½ cup strawberry preserves
- 1 tablespoon cornstarch dissolved in 2 tablespoons water

DIRECTIONS

1   Make the crust: In a food processor, combine the flour, salt, and sugar and pulse to combine. Add the margarine and process until crumbly. With the machine running, stream in the water and process to form a soft dough. Do not overmix. Flatten the dough into a disk and wrap it in plastic wrap.

2   Refrigerate for 30 minutes. Preheat the oven to 400°F.

3   Roll out the dough on a lightly floured work surface to about 10 inches in diameter. Fit the dough into a 9-inch pie plate. Trim and flute the edges. Prick holes in the bottom of the dough with a fork. Bake for 10 minutes, then remove from the oven and set aside. Reduce the oven temperature to 350°F.

4   Make the filling: In a blender or food processor, combine the tofu, sugar, and vanilla and blend until smooth. Pour into the prepared crust.

5   Bake for 30 minutes. Remove from the oven and set aside to cool for 30 minutes.

6   Arrange the sliced strawberries on top of the pie in a decorative pattern to cover the entire surface. Set aside.

7   Puree the preserves in a blender or food processor and transfer to a small saucepan over medium heat. Stir in the cornstarch mixture and continue stirring until the mixture has thickened.

8   Spoon the strawberry glaze over the pie. Refrigerate the pie at least 1 hour before serving to chill the filling and set the glaze.

MEDITERRANEAN
SEAFOOD

Pan-seared salmon with zucchini pesto

SERVES: 4

INGREDIENTS

Zucchini Pasto

- 3 ripe medium-sized tomatoes, cored and quartered
- 2 tablespoons extra-virgin olive oil (preferably Spanish olive oil)
- 1 medium yellow onion, finely chopped
- 1 garlic clove, very finely chopped
- 1 red bell pepper--halved, seeded, and chopped into ¼-inch pieces
- 2 medium zucchini, ends trimmed and zucchini chopped into ¼-inch pieces
- 1 sprig of fresh rosemary
- 1 sprig of fresh thyme
- 1 teaspoon kosher salt

Salmon

- Four 6- to 8-ounce salmon fillets, pin bones removed
- 1 teaspoon kosher salt
- 1 teaspoon freshly ground black pepper
- 1 tablespoon extra-virgin olive oil (preferably Spanish olive oil)

DIRECTIONS

1 Make the zucchini pesto: To a blender, add the tomato quarters and purée until smooth. Set aside.

2   In a large skillet set over medium-high heat, add the 2 tablespoons olive oil and the onion. Cook, stirring often, until the onion is translucent, 2 to 3 minutes.

3   Add the garlic and stir until fragrant, about 30 seconds. Reduce the heat to medium-low and add the red bell pepper, stirring occasionally, until it begins to soften about 10 minutes. Stir in the zucchini and cook until it begins to soften for about 8 minutes.

4   Add the blended tomatoes and simmer on low heat until the pesto looks thick and has reduced by half, about 35 minutes.

5   Add the rosemary and thyme sprigs and simmer for 5 minutes. Turn off the heat and discard the rosemary and thyme. Season with 1 teaspoon of salt.

6   Cook the salmon: Use paper towels to pat both sides of each salmon fillet dry. Season the fillets with 1 teaspoon of salt and black pepper. In a large skillet set over high heat, add 1 tablespoon of olive oil.

7   Once the oil begins to shimmer, add 2 of the salmon fillets, skin side down. Cook the salmon without moving the fillets until the skin is browned, about 4 minutes.

8   Use a fish spatula to gently flip each fillet over, and cook until the center of the fillets are semi-firm, about 3 minutes more. Transfer to a plate and repeat with the remaining 2 salmon fillets. Serve with the zucchini pesto.

Poached Salmon in Tomato Garlic Broth

Serves: 4

INGREDIENTS

- 8 cloves garlic
- shallots
- teaspoons extra virgin olive oil
- 5 ripe tomatoes
- 1 1/2 cups dry white wine
- 1 cup water
- 8 sprigs of thyme 1/4 teaspoon sea salt
- 1/4 teaspoon fresh black pepper
- 4 Copper River Sockeye Salmon fillets white truffle oil (optional)

DIRECTIONS

1   Peel and roughly chop garlic cloves and shallots. In a large braising dish or sauté pan with a lid, place the olive oil, garlic, and shallots. Sweat over medium-low heat until soft, about 3 minutes.

2   Place the tomatoes, wine, water, thyme, salt, and pepper in the pan and bring to a boil. Once boiling, reduce heat to a simmer and cover.

3   Simmer for 25 minutes until the tomatoes have burst to release their juices. With a wooden spoon or spatula, crush the tomatoes into a pulp. Simmer uncovered for another 5 minutes until the broth has reduced a little.

4   While the broth is still simmering, place the salmon in the broth. Cover and poach for 5 to 6 minutes only until the fish easily flakes.

5   Place the fish on a plate and set it aside. Place a strainer into a large bowl and pour the remaining broth into the strainer. Strain the broth discarding the solids that remain. Taste the broth and add salt and pepper if needed.

6   Simple butter mashed potatoes or even roasted potatoes are a good side of this meal. To plate, place mashed potatoes in a large bowl or a deep plate. Then top with sauteed asparagus and the poached salmon. Pour the strained broth around the salmon. Add a drizzle of white truffle oil if desired. Serve.

Prosciutto/Salmon Wraps

SERVES: 8

INGREDIENTS

- avocados, seeded and peeled
- slices each prosciutto and smoked salmon Fresh lemon or lime
- Cut each avocado into 8 slices. Diagonally wrap each with a prosciutto or salmon slice. Arrange wraps on a serving platter, garnish with lemon or lime and serve.

Salmon Croquettes

- oz. Can of red or pink salmon, drained
- 1 Small onion, finely chopped
- 1 Teaspoon Fresh lemon juice
- 1 Egg, lightly beaten
- 12−15 Saltine crackers, crushed
- ¼ Teaspoon Ground pepper
- Teaspoon Fresh parsley, chopped (optional)
- ¼ Cup Canola oil

DIRECTIONS

1 Mash drained salmon in a bowl. Add chopped onion, lemon juice, egg, pepper, and, if desired, parsley. Mix gently. Shape into six croquettes (patties).

2   Crush the saltines between two sheets of waxed paper with a rolling pin. Set each croquette into the crumbs, pressing gently to make sure crumbs adhere, turning to coat both sides.

3   Heat oil in a skillet over medium heat. Fry croquettes on one side until golden brown, then gently turn and fry the other side. Serves 4 to 6, depending upon appetites.

Salmon Pate

SERVES: 4

INGREDIENTS

- 1 cup salmon, flaked
- 1 pkg. (8 oz.) cream cheese, room temperature
- 1 tablespoon fresh lemon juice
- 1 teaspoon prepared horseradish
- 1 teaspoon onion, grated
- 1/4 teaspoon salt
- 1/8 teaspoon pepper
- 1/8 teaspoon liquid smoke

Garnish:
- almond slices
- parsley
- Olives
- Celery

DIRECTIONS

1 Mix Salmon with all of the other ingredients. Press into a fish-shaped mold or shape by hand as such.
2 Garnish fish with almond slices to resemble scales.
3 Slice green olive for the eye and thin strips of celery for the tail.
4 Garnish top with parsley. Chill at least 1 hour before serving.

Spice-Rubbed Salmon with Sautéed Greens

SERVES: 4

INGREDIENTS

- 4 4-ounce salmon fillets*
- 1 tablespoon fennel seeds
- 1 teaspoon coriander seeds
- 1 tablespoon lemon juice
- 2 tablespoons olive oil
- salt and pepper, to taste
- lemon or lime slices (optional)

DIRECTIONS

1. We used salmon steaks, which we cut in half and deboned. You can choose to keep the skin off or remove it before cooking.

2. Rinse the salmon fillets and trim/debone if necessary. Place in a large bowl.

3. Using a spice grinder or mortar and pestle, coarsely grind the coriander and fennel seeds together

4. Add the seeds, salt and pepper, lemon juice, and oil to the fish and rub the spices into each side of the salmon fillets. Let sit for a few minutes as you turn your oven's broiler to high.

5. Place the fish on a lined baking sheet, topping with lemon or lime slices if desired. Broil for 6 minutes, turning halfway.

6. **For the greens:**

7   tablespoons olive oil

8   1 clove garlic, sliced

9   ounces mixed greens, such as spinach, chard, and dandelion (we used a Satur Farms stir-fry blend), trimmed and rinsed

10   1 teaspoon crushed red pepper

11   salt and pepper, to taste

12   Heat the oil on medium in a large skillet.

13   Add the garlic and saute until slightly browned. Add the greens, crushed red pepper, salt, and pepper, and saute until the greens are wilted for about 5 minutes.

Smoked Salmon and Scrambled Eggs

SERVES: 2

INGREDIENTS

- fresh eggs
- Knob of butter
- 150g pack of smoked salmon
- Salt and pepper
- slices Sourdough bread

DIRECTIONS

1   Pre-heat griddle pan. Heat your non-stick pan gently and add a knob of the butter. And add your beaten eggs. Gently cook and stir.

2   Continue to cook for a couple of minutes, whilst still just underdone. Griddle the bread until nicely charred on each side.

3   When the eggs thicken, season with salt and pepper and pile the eggs over the toast. Top with smoked salmon slices.

4   Serve with a good wedge of lemon and freshly ground black pepper.

Stovetop Smoked Salmon with Dill-Lemon Aioli

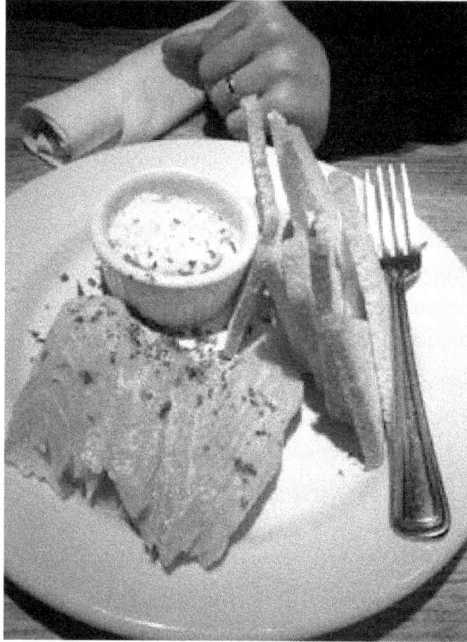

SERVES: 4

INGREDIENTS

- smoking chips
- 1-1/2 lb. fresh boneless salmon filet, about 1-inch thick
- juice of 1/2 lime
- Tbsp. white wine
- 1 Tbsp. mayonnaise
- 1/2 tsp. kosher salt
- 1/2 tsp. onion powder
- 1/2 tsp. garlic powder

- 1/2 tsp. lemon pepper
- 1/2 tsp. dried oregano
- 1/2 tsp. dried dill weed
- 1/4 tsp. paprika

DIRECTIONS

1   Sprinkle smoking chips over the bottom of the smoker. Place drip pan over chips. (Line drip pan with foil for easier clean-up, but make sure the foil is pressed tightly to the pan so you don't disrupt the air-flow of the smoke.) Brush the wire grill rack with vegetable oil and place it in the drip pan. Place fish on rack.

2   Squeeze lime over salmon. Drizzle with wine. Combine remaining ingredients, brush the mixture onto the top of the fish.

3   Position smoker over one stovetop burner as evenly as possible. Heat smoker on medium-high and offset lid so it is not tightly closed. When wisps of smoke begin to come through the opening, re-position the lid so it is tightly closed.

4   Cook 15 to 25 min., depending on the thickness of the fish. The fish should just barely give to the touch, like a medium-cooked steak. Let rest 5 min. before serving with aioli.

Dill-Lemon Aioli

SERVES: 4

INGREDIENTS

- egg yolks
- 1/2 tsp. lemon zest
- 1/4 cup lemon juice
- garlic cloves, minced
- 1-1/2 tsp. chopped fresh parsley
- 1 tsp. kosher salt
- 3/4 tsp. dried dill weed
- 1/4 tsp. Worcestershire sauce
- 1/8 tsp. cayenne pepper
- 3/4 cup olive oil

DIRECTIONS

1   Place all ingredients, except oil, in a blender. Pulse to combine.

2   With blender running, very slowly drizzle in olive oil, little by little, until an emulsion forms (the mixture will thicken and become a creamy, white color).

3   Refrigerate 1 hour before serving to allow flavors to combine.

Soy-Ginger Marinated Salmon

SERVES: 4

INGREDIENTS

- salmon fillets or steaks (allow about 6 oz. per person)
- Marinade (see the following recipe)
- Lemon wedges, optional
  Marinade:
- 1 cup sake (Japanese rice wine)
- 1/2 cup natural soy sauce or tamari (preferably reduced sodium)
- 1 tbsp. freshly grated ginger
- cloves fresh garlic, pressed
- 1 tablespoon dark brown sugar

DIRECTIONS

1 Make the marinade by whisking the marinade ingredients together in a small bowl.

2 Rinse the salmon fillets under cold water, and place in a glass or ceramic dish. Pour the marinade over the fish.

3 Cover the dish and allow the fish to marinate in the refrigerator for several hours (about one to three hours). At least once or twice during this time, check the fish and spoon the marinade over any exposed parts of the fillets.

4 Fire the grill, or preheat the broiler to high heat.

5   Drain the fish and place it on foil on a grill or rack in the oven. Cook until desired doneness, (fish flakes easily and is opaque) but be careful not to overcook.

6   Serve immediately, with lemon wedges as garnish if you like. For a complete, satisfying meal, add rice and a salad or steamed vegetables.

Sweet Salmon with Ginger and Scallions

SERVES: 2

INGREDIENTS

- (1–inch thick) salmon filets
- scallions, cut into 2–inch long strips
- 1/4 cup ginger, cut into 1/4–inch thick chunks
- 1 1/2 tablespoons olive oil
- 1/4 cup white wine, rice wine, or sweet sake
- 1/2 cup water
- 1 tablespoon soy sauce
- 1 teaspoon granulated sugar
- Salt and pepper
- Sesame oil (optional)

DIRECTIONS

Heat oil in a pan on high heat. Salt and pepper on both sides of the salmon filets.
Place filets in pan skin–side down and do not disturb. Cook on high for 40 sec.
Turn heat down to medium–high and continue to cook for 3 minutes.

Turn filets over and cook for another 2 minutes. Remove filets from the pan and
set them aside on a plate.

Turn the heat back up to high and add ginger and scallions. Cook until slightly tender (about 1 minute). Add wine and deglaze the pan. Add soy sauce, water, and sugar. Bring to a boil, then reduce heat to simmer.

Place salmon filets carefully back into the pan and simmer until salmon is cooked through (about 2 minutes). Drizzle with a few drops of sesame oil if desired.

Butter Barbecued Salmon

SERVES: 4

INGREDIENTS

- 6--8 lb whole salmon, cleaned
- salt & pepper, to taste
- cups chopped mushrooms
- 1 cup chopped green onions
- tbs minced parsley
- 1/2 cup grated Parmesan cheese Grated peel and juice of 1 lemon
- 1/2 cup (1 stick) butter or margarine, melted 4-5 lemon slices
- sauces: butter, chili-cheese, or tartar

DIRECTIONS

1   Remove head from salmon, if desired. Place salmon on a double thickness of wide foil, making sure foil is three to four inches longer than fish at each end. Sprinkle fish inside and out with salt and pepper to taste. Combine mushrooms, onion, parsley, cheese, lemon peel, and juice.

2   Spoon mixture into the fish cavity. Pour butter over fish and top with lemon slices. Cover with another thickness of foil and carefully seal all sides completely. Place on grill four to six inches from glowing coals. Turn after 30 minutes and cook 20 to 30 minutes longer. If cooking on the smoke-type grill, open foil during the last ten minutes and close grill cover so smoke flavor penetrates fish. Serve with a choice of sauces. Makes 10 to 12 servings.

Butter Sauce

- 1/2 cup butter or margarine
- 1 cup sour cream
- 1/4 tsp seasoned or onion salt
- 1 tsp chopped chives

DIRECTIONS

1 Melt butter in a small saucepan over low heat.
2 Stir in sour cream, seasoned salt, and chives.
3 Warm, but do not boil.

Curried Salmon-Rice Loaf

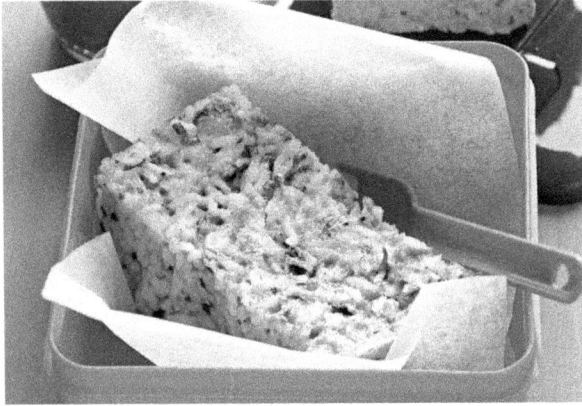

SERVES: 2

INGREDIENTS

- 1 can (17 1/2 ounce) salmon
- 1/3 cup chopped green onions
- tsp curry powder
- 1 tbs lemon juice
- 1 tbs cider vinegar
- 1 tbs chopped or powdered garlic
- cups cooked rice
- Lettuce

DIRECTIONS

1 Flake salmon.

2 Remove skin and bones.

3 Add salmon, green onions, curry powder, lemon juice, cider vinegar, and garlic to rice. Mix well. Pack into plastic-lined loaf pan and chill several hours in the refrigerator. When ready to serve, unmold onto a lettuce-lined platter. Makes 4 servings.

Salmon-Broccoli Loaf with Dill and Capers

SERVES: 4

INGREDIENTS

1 c loosely packed parsley sprigs, washed & patted dry on paper towels

6 slices firm-textured white bread

2 c 1/2 inch cubes of broccoli stems (the amt you'll get from one large bunch of broccoli. Amount can be variable.)

1 medium yellow onion, cut into slim wedges

1 3/4 pounds cooked or canned boned salmon (remove all dark skin)

1/3 c drained capers (use the small capers)

2/3 c light cream

4 eggs

2 TBS snipped fresh dill or 3/4 tsp dill weed Finely grated rind of 1/2 lemon 1/8 tsp freshly ground black pepper

DIRECTIONS

1   In a food processor fitted with a metal chopping blade, mince parsley fine, using 5-6 on-offs of the motor; empty into a large mixing bowl. Now crumb the bread 2 slices at a time, with two or three 5-or 6 churnings of the motor; add to bowl.

2   Dump all the broccoli stems into processor; mince very fine with about three 5-second bursts; add to bowl.

3   Processor-mince the onion -- 3 o4 4 bursts will do it -- add to the bowl.

4   Flake the salmon in three batches - 2 on-offs will be enough.

5   Add to the mixing bowl along with all remaining ingredients.

89

6   Mix v thoroughly, pack mixture firmly into a well-buttered 9x5x3 inch loaf pan, and bake in a slow oven (300 degrees F.) for about 1 hour and 40 minutes, or until loaf begins to pull from sides of the pan and is firm to the touch.

7   Remove loaf from the oven and let it stand upright in its pan on a wire rack for 30 minutes. Carefully loosen the loaf all around w a thin-bladed spatula, then invert gently onto a large serving platter.

Salmon in Vodka Cream Sauce with Green Peppercorns

SERVES: 4

INGREDIENTS

- tablespoons butter
- 1 onion, thinly sliced
- 1 pound spinach
- 6 ounce salmon filets
- salt and freshly ground pepper
- tablespoons olive oil
- 1 1/2 cups whipping cream
- 1/2 cup vodka
- tablespoons green peppercorns in water, drained and crushed
- tablespoons fresh lime juice
- 1/4 cup snipped fresh chives

DIRECTIONS

1   Preheat oven to 350F. Combine 4 tablespoons of butter and onion in a large Dutch oven. Cover and bake until onion is golden brown, stirring occasionally, about 45 minutes.

2   Stir spinach into the onion and bake until just wilted about 3 minutes.

3   Remove from oven; keep warm.

4   Season salmon with salt and pepper. Heat oil in a heavy large skillet over high heat. Add salmon in batches and cook for about 3 minutes per side for medium. Transfer to a platter. Tent with foil to keep warm. Pour off excess oil from the skillet.

5   Add cream and vodka and boil until slightly thickened, about 4 minutes. Add green peppercorns and the remaining 4 tablespoons of butter and stir until butter is just melted. Mix in lime juice, season with salt and pepper.

6   Divide spinach and onion mixture among plates. Top each with a salmon fillet. Spoon sauce over. Sprinkle with snipped fresh chives.

MEDITERRANEAN PASTA

Saucy Cheddar Fusilli Salad

PREP TIME: 15 Minutes

COOKING TIME: 90 Minutes

SERVES 10

INGREDIENTS

- 2 tbsp olive oil
- 6 green onions, chopped
- 1 tsp salt
- 3/4 C. chopped pickled jalapeno peppers
- 1 (16 oz) package fusilli pasta
- 1 (2.25 oz) can slice black olives
- 2 lb. extra lean ground beef
- (optional)
- 1 (1.25 oz) package taco seasoning mix
- 1 (8 oz) package shredded Cheddar
- 1 (24 oz) jar mild salsa
- cheese
- 1 (8 oz) bottle ranch dressing
- 1 1/2 red bell peppers, chopped

DIRECTIONS

1. Place a large pot over medium heat. Fill it with water and stir into it the olive oil with salt.

Cook it until it starts boiling.

2. Add the pasta and boil it for 10 min. Remove it from the water and place it aside to drain.

3. Place a large pan over medium heat. Brown in it the beef for 12 min. Discard the excess grease.

4. Add the taco seasoning and mix them well. Place the mix aside to lose heat completely.

5. Get a large mixing bowl: Mix in it the salsa, ranch dressing, bell peppers, green onions, jalapenos, and black olives.

6. Add the pasta with cooked beef, Cheddar cheese, and dressing mix. Stir them well. Place a piece of plastic wrap over the salad bowl. Place it in the fridge for 1 h 15 min.

NUTRITIONAL VALUES

Calories 597 kcal, Fat 34 g, Carbohydrates 43.2g, Protein 29.9 g

Creamy Penn Pasta Salad

PREP TIME: 20 Minutes

COOKING TIME: 150 Minutes

SERVES 10

INGREDIENTS

- 1 (16 oz) box mini penne pasta
- 1/3 C. chopped red onion
- 1 1/2 lb. chopped cooked chicken
- 1/2 (8 oz) bottle creamy Caesar salad dressing, 1/2 C. diced green bell pepper
- or to taste
- 2 hard-boiled eggs, chopped
- 1/3 C. grated Parmesan cheese

DIRECTIONS

1   Cook the pasta according to the directions on the package.
2   Get a large mixing bowl: Toss in it the pasta, chicken, green bell pepper, eggs, Parmesan cheese, and red onion.
3   Add the dressing and stir them well. Cover the bowl and place it in the fridge for 2 h 15 min. Adjust the seasoning of the salad and serve it.
4   Enjoy.

NUTRITIONAL VALUES

Calories 381 kcal, Fat 15.5 g, Carbohydrates 34.1g, Protein 25.5 g, Cholesterol 102 mg, Sodium 210 mg

Italian Dessert Noodles

PREP TIME: 10 Minutes

COOKING TIME: 60 Minutes

SERVES 15

INGREDIENTS

- 1 (12 oz.) package wide egg noodles
- 1 tsp salt
- 1/2 C. butter, melted
- 4 eggs, beaten
- 3/4 C. white sugar
- 1/4 tsp ground cinnamon
- 3/4 C. raisins
- 3/4 C. coarsely chopped pecans

DIRECTIONS

1. Set your oven to 375 degrees F before doing anything else and grease a 12x8-inch baking dish with some melted butter evenly.
2. In a large pan of lightly salted boiling water, cook the egg noodles for about 8-10 minutes.
3. Drain well.

4. In a large bowl, mix the remaining butter, noodles, eggs, pecans, raisins, sugar, and salt.

5. Transfer the mixture into the prepared baking dish and sprinkle it with cinnamon.

6. Cook everything in the oven for about 55 minutes.

NUTRITIONAL VALUES

Calories 243 kcal, Fat 12.6 g, Carbohydrates 29.1g, Protein 4.9 g, Cholesterol 82 mg, Sodium 221 mg

Egg Noodles Hungarian

PREP TIME: 15 Minutes

COOKING TIME: 50 Minutes

SERVES 6

INGREDIENTS

- 1 (8 oz.) package fine egg noodles
- 2 tbsp poppy seeds
- 2 C. cottage cheese
- 1 tsp salt
- 2 C. sour cream
- 1 tbsp grated Parmesan cheese
- 1/2 C. chopped onions
- 1 pinch ground paprika
- 2 tbsp Worcestershire sauce

DIRECTIONS

1. Set your oven to 350 degrees F before doing anything else and grease a large casserole dish.
2. In a large pan of lightly salted boiling water, cook the egg noodles for about 5 minutes, stirring occasionally.
3. Drain them well and keep everything aside.
4. In a large bowl, add the noodles and remaining ingredients except the Parmesan cheese and paprika and mix well.

5. Transfer the mixture into the prepared casserole dish evenly and top with Parmesan cheese and paprika.
6. Cook everything in the oven for about 30 minutes

NUTRITIONAL VALUES

Calories 414 kcal, Fat 22.6 g, Carbohydrates 35.1g, Protein 18.1 g, Cholesterol 77 mg, Sodium 809 mg

Pennsylvanian Noodles

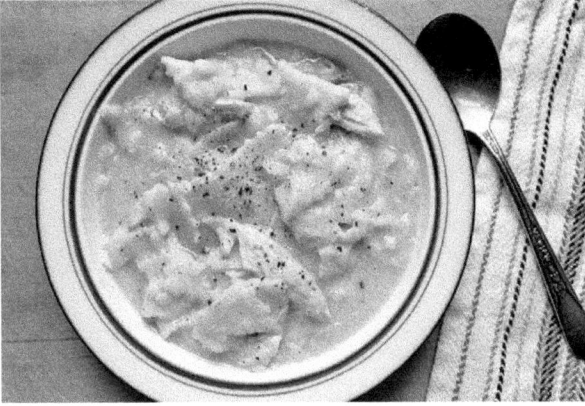

PREP TIME: 5 Minutes

COOKING TIME: 15 Minutes

SERVES 4

INGREDIENTS

- 8 oz. wide egg noodles
- 1/4-1/2 C. salted butter

DIRECTIONS

1. In a large pan of boiling water, prepare the egg noodles according to the package's directions.
2. Drain well and transfer into a large bowl.

3. Meanwhile, in a small frying pan, add the butter and melt, stirring till the butter starts to become brown.

4. Pour melted butter, salt, and black pepper and stir to coat well.

NUTRITIONAL VALUES

Calories 320.6, Fat 14.0g, Cholesterol 78.3mg, Sodium 113.2mg, Carbohydrates 40.6g, Protein 8.1g

VEGAN MAIN DISHES

Millet and Amaranth Loaf

SERVES: 4

INGREDIENTS

- 2 cups vegetable broth, homemade (see Light Vegetable Broth) or store-bought, or water ¾ cup millet
- ¼ cup amaranth
- Salt
- 1 medium yellow onion, finely chopped
- 2 garlic cloves, minced
- 1 medium zucchini, finely chopped
- ½ cup frozen peas
- ¼ cup minced fresh parsley
- 1 teaspoon dried thyme
- Freshly ground black pepper

DIRECTIONS

1. In a large saucepan, bring the broth to a boil over high heat.
2. Add the millet, amaranth, and salt to taste. Cook until the grains are soft and the water is absorbed about 25 minutes.
3. Preheat the oven to 350°F. Lightly oil a 9-inch loaf pan and set it aside. In a large skillet, heat the oil over medium heat.

4. Add the onion, cover, and cook until soft, about 8 minutes. Add the garlic, zucchini, and peas and cook until the vegetables are softened. Add the parsley, thyme, and salt and pepper to taste.

5. Stir in the cooked millet and amaranth, then transfer the mixture to the prepared loaf pan. Bake until golden brown on top, about 20 minutes. Serve immediately.

Savory Amaranth Patties

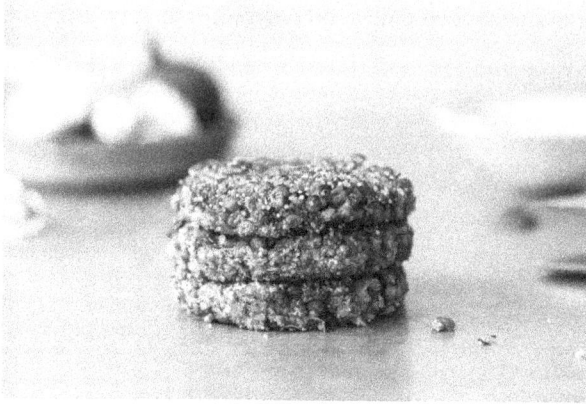

SERVES: 4

INGREDIENTS

- 1 cup water
- ½ cup amaranth
- Salt
- 2 tablespoons olive oil
- ½ cup minced onion
- ½ cup shredded carrot
- ½ cup ground walnuts
- 1 teaspoon soy sauce
- 2 tablespoons wheat gluten flour (vital wheat gluten)
- 2 tablespoons minced fresh parsley or cilantro
- Freshly ground black pepper

DIRECTIONS

1. In a small saucepan, bring the water to a boil over high heat. Add the amaranth and salt to taste and reduce the heat to low. Cover and simmer until the amaranth is cooked, about 15 to 20 minutes. Set aside.

2. In a large skillet, heat 1 tablespoon of the oil over medium heat.

3. Add the onion and carrot. Cover and cook until soft, 5 minutes. Stir in the walnuts and cook, uncovered, 2 minutes longer. Transfer the mixture to a large bowl. Add the soy sauce, flour, parsley, and salt and pepper to taste. Add the cooked amaranth and stir to mix well.

4. Form the mixture into 4 patties. Heat the remaining 2 tablespoons of oil in a large nonstick skillet. Add the patties and cook until browned on both sides, turning once about 10 minutes total. Serve immediately.

Soy-Glazed Tofu

SERVES: 4

INGREDIENTS

- 1 pound extra-firm tofu, drained, cut into ½-inch slices, and pressed
- ¼ cup toasted sesame oil
- ¼ cup rice vinegar
- 2 teaspoons sugar

DIRECTIONS

Blot the tofu dry and arrange in a 9 x 13inch baking dish and set aside.

In a small saucepan, combine the soy sauce, oil, vinegar, and sugar and bring to a boil. Pour the hot marinade onto the tofu and set aside to marinate for 30 minutes, turning once.

Preheat the oven to 350°F. Bake the tofu for 30 minutes, turning once about halfway through.

Serve immediately or allow to cool to room temperature, then cover and refrigerate until needed.

Cajun-Style Tofu

SERVES: 4

INGREDIENTS

- 1 pound extra-firm tofu, drained and patted dry
- Salt
- 1 tablespoon plus 1 teaspoon Cajun seasoning
- 2 tablespoons olive oil
- ¼ cup minced green bell pepper
- 1 tablespoon minced celery
- 2 tablespoons minced green onion
- 2 garlic cloves, minced
- 1 (14.5-ounce) can diced tomatoes, drained
- 1 tablespoon soy sauce
- 1 tablespoon minced fresh parsley

DIRECTIONS

1. Cut the tofu into ½-inch thick slices and sprinkle both sides with salt and the 1 tablespoon Cajun seasoning. Set aside.
2. In a small saucepan, heat 1 tablespoon of the oil over medium heat.
3. Add the bell pepper and celery. Cover and cook for 5 minutes. Add the green onion and garlic and cook, uncovered, 1 minute longer.

4. Stir in the tomatoes, soy sauce, parsley, the remaining 1 teaspoon Cajun spice blend, and salt to taste. Simmer for 10 minutes to blend the flavors and set aside.

5. In a large skillet, heat the remaining 1 tablespoon oil over medium-high heat. Add the tofu and cook until browned on both sides, about 10 minutes.

6. Add the sauce and simmer for 5 minutes. Serve immediately.

Crispy Tofu with Sizzling Caper Sauce

SERVES: 4

INGREDIENTS

- 1 pound extra-firm tofu, drained, cut into ¼-inch slices, and pressed
- Salt and freshly ground black pepper
- 2 tablespoons olive oil, plus more if needed
- 1 medium shallot, minced
- 2 tablespoons capers
- 3 tablespoons minced fresh parsley
- 2 tablespoons vegan margarine
- Juice of 1 lemon

DIRECTIONS

1. Preheat the oven to 275°F. Pat the tofu dry and season with salt and pepper to taste. Place the cornstarch in a shallow bowl. Dredge the tofu in the cornstarch, coating all sides.

2. In a large skillet, heat 2 tablespoons of the oil over medium heat.

3. Add the tofu, in batches if necessary, and cook until golden brown on both sides, about 4 minutes per side. Transfer the fried tofu to a heatproof platter and keep warm in the oven.

4. In the same skillet, heat the remaining 1 tablespoon of the oil over medium heat. Add the shallot and cook until softened, about 3 minutes.

5. Add the capers and parsley and cook for 30 seconds, then stir in the margarine, lemon juice, and salt and pepper to taste, stirring to melt and incorporate the margarine.
6. Top the tofu with caper sauce and serve immediately.

Country-Fried Tofu with Golden Gravy

SERVES: 4

INGREDIENTS

- 1 pound extra-firm tofu, drained, cut into ½-inch slices, and pressed
- Salt and freshly ground black pepper
- ⅓ cup cornstarch
- 2 tablespoons olive oil
- 1 medium sweet yellow onion, chopped
- 2 tablespoons all-purpose flour
- 1 teaspoon dried thyme
- ⅛ teaspoon turmeric
- 1 cup vegetable broth, homemade (see Light Vegetable Broth) or store-bought
- 1 tablespoon soy sauce
- 1 cup cooked or canned chickpeas, drained and rinsed
- 2 tablespoons minced fresh parsley, for garnish

DIRECTIONS

1. Blot the tofu dry and season with salt and pepper to taste. Place the cornstarch in a shallow bowl. Dredge the tofu in the cornstarch, coating all sides. Preheat the oven to 250°F.
2. In a large skillet, heat 2 tablespoons of the oil over medium heat.

3. Add the tofu, in batches if necessary, and cook until golden brown on both sides, about 10 minutes. Transfer the fried tofu to a heatproof platter and keep warm in the oven.

4. In the same skillet, heat the remaining 1 tablespoon of the oil over medium heat. Add the onion, cover, and cook until softened, 5 minutes.

5. Uncover and reduce heat to low. Stir in the flour, thyme, and turmeric and cook for 1 minute, stirring constantly. Slowly whisk in the broth, then the soy milk and soy sauce. Add the chickpeas and season with salt and pepper to taste.

6. Continue to cook, stir frequently, for 2 minutes. Transfer to a blender and process until smooth and creamy. Return to the saucepan and heat until hot, adding a little more broth if the sauce is too thick. Spoon the sauce over the tofu and sprinkle with the parsley. Serve immediately.

Orange-Glazed Tofu and Asparagus

SERVES: 4

INGREDIENTS

- 2 tablespoons mirin
- 1 tablespoon cornstarch
- 1 (16-ounce) package extra-firm tofu, drained, and cut into ¼-inch strips
- 2 tablespoons soy sauce
- 1 teaspoon toasted sesame oil
- 1 teaspoon sugar
- ¼ teaspoon Asian chili paste
- 2 tablespoons canola or grapeseed oil
- 1 garlic clove, minced
- ½ teaspoon minced fresh ginger
- 5 ounces thin asparagus, tough ends trimmed and cut into 1½-inch pieces

DIRECTIONS

1. In a shallow bowl, combine the mirin and cornstarch and blend well. Add the tofu and toss gently to the coat. Set aside to marinate for 30 minutes.
2. In a small bowl, combine the orange juice, soy sauce, sesame oil, sugar, and chili paste. Set aside.
3. In a large skillet or wok, heat the canola oil over medium heat. Add the garlic and ginger and stir-fry until fragrant, about 30 seconds.

4. Add the marinated tofu and the asparagus and stir-fry until the tofu is golden brown and the asparagus is just tender about 5 minutes.

5. Stir in the sauce and cook for about 2 minutes more. Serve immediately.

Tofu Pizzaiola

SERVES: 4

INGREDIENTS

- 2 tablespoons olive oil
- 1 (16-ounce) package extra-firm tofu, drained, cut into ½-inch slices, and pressed (see Light Vegetable Broth)
- Salt
- 3 garlic cloves, minced
- 1 (14.5-ounce) can diced tomatoes, drained
- ¼ cup oil-packed sun-dried tomatoes, cut into ¼-inch strips
- 1 tablespoon capers
- 1 teaspoon dried oregano
- ½ teaspoon sugar
- Freshly ground black pepper
- 2 tablespoons minced fresh parsley, for garnish

DIRECTIONS

1. Preheat the oven to 275°F. In a large skillet, heat 1 tablespoon of the oil over medium heat.
2. Add the tofu and cook until golden brown on both sides, turning once, about 5 minutes per side. Sprinkle the tofu with salt to taste.
3. Transfer the fried tofu to a heatproof platter and keep warm in the oven.

4. In the same skillet, heat the remaining 1 tablespoon oil over medium heat. Add the garlic and cook until softened, about 1 minute.

5. Do not brown. Stir in the diced tomatoes, sun-dried tomatoes, olives, and capers. Add the oregano, sugar, and salt, and pepper to taste.

6. Simmer until the sauce is hot and the flavors are well combined about 10 minutes.

7. Top the fried tofu slices with the sauce and sprinkle with the parsley. Serve immediately.

Ka-Pow Tofu

SERVES: 4

INGREDIENTS

- 1 pound extra-firm tofu, drained, patted dry, and cut into 1-inch cubes
- Salt
- 2 tablespoons cornstarch
- 2 tablespoons soy sauce
- 1 tablespoon vegetarian oyster sauce
- 2 teaspoons Nothin' Fishy Nam Pla (see Nothin' Fishy Nam Pla) or 1 teaspoon rice vinegar
- 1 teaspoon light brown sugar
- ½ teaspoon crushed red pepper
- 2 tablespoons canola or grapeseed oil
- 1 medium sweet yellow onion, halved and cut into ½-inch slices
- medium red bell pepper, cut into ¼-inch slices
- green onions, chopped
- ½ cup Thai basil leaves

DIRECTIONS

1. In a medium bowl, combine the tofu, salt to taste, and cornstarch. Toss to coat and set aside.
2. In a small bowl, combine the soy sauce, oyster sauce, nam pla, sugar, and crushed red pepper. Stir well to combine and set aside.

119

3. In a large skillet, heat 1 tablespoon of the oil over medium-high heat. Add the tofu and cook until golden brown, about 8 minutes.

4. Remove from the skillet and set aside.

5. In the same skillet, heat the remaining 1 tablespoon oil over medium heat. Add the onion and bell pepper and stir-fry until softened, about 5 minutes.

6. Add the green onions and cook 1 minute longer. Stir in the fried tofu, the sauce, and the basil and stir-fry until hot, about 3 minutes. Serve immediately.

Sicilian-Style Tofu

SERVES: 4

INGREDIENTS

- 2 tablespoons olive oil
- 1 pound extra-firm tofu, drained, cut into ¼-inch slices, and pressed Salt and freshly ground black pepper
- 1 small yellow onion, chopped
- 2 garlic cloves, minced
- 1 (28-ounce) can diced tomatoes, drained
- ¼ cup dry white wine
- ¼ teaspoon crushed red pepper
- ⅓ cup pitted Kalamata olives
- 1½ tablespoons capers
- 2 tablespoons chopped fresh basil or 1 teaspoon dried (optional)

DIRECTIONS

1. Preheat the oven to 250°F. In a large skillet, heat 1 tablespoon of the oil over medium heat.
2. Add the tofu, in batches if necessary, and cook until golden brown on both sides, 5 minutes per side. Season with salt and black pepper to taste.
3. Transfer the cooked tofu to a heatproof platter and keep warm in the oven while you prepare the sauce.

4. In the same skillet, heat the remaining 1 tablespoon oil over medium heat. Add the onion and garlic, cover, and cook until the onion is softened, 10 minutes. Add the tomatoes, wine, and crushed red pepper.

5. Bring to a boil, then reduce heat to low and simmer, uncovered, for 15 minutes. Stir in the olives and capers. Cook for 2 minutes more.

6. Arrange the tofu on a platter or individual plates. Spoon the sauce on top.

7. Sprinkle with fresh basil, if using. Serve immediately.

COOKING CONVERSION CHART

TEMPERATURE		WEIGHT	
FAHRENHEIT	CELSIUS	IMPERIAL	METRIC
100 °F	37 °C	1/2 oz	15 g
150 °F	65 °C	1 oz	29 g
200 °F	93 °C	2 oz	57 g
250 °F	121 °C	3 oz	85 g
300 °F	150 °C	4 oz	113 g
325 °F	160 °C	5 oz	141 g
350 °F	180 °C	6 oz	170 g
375 °F	190 °C	8 oz	227 g
400 °F	200 °C	10 oz	283 g
425 °F	220 °C	12 oz	340 g
450 °F	230 °C	13 oz	369 g
500 °F	260 °C	14 oz	397 g
525 °F	270 °C	15 oz	425 g
550 °F	288 °C	1 lb	453 g

MEASUREMENT			
CUP	ONCES	MILLILITERS	TABLESPOON
1/16 cup	1/2 oz	15 ml	1
1/8 cup	1 oz	30 ml	3
1/4 cup	2 oz	59 ml	4
1/3 cup	2.5 oz	79 ml	5.5
3/8 cup	3 oz	90 ml	6
1/2 cup	4 oz	118 ml	8
2/3 cup	5 oz	158 ml	11
3/4 cup	6 oz	177 ml	12
1 cup	8 oz	240 ml	16
2 cup	16 oz	480 ml	32
4 cup	32 oz	960 ml	64
5 cup	40 oz	1180 ml	80
6 cup	48 oz	1420 ml	96
8 cup	64 oz	1895 ml	128

Lightning Source UK Ltd.
Milton Keynes UK
UKHW021835040621
384966UK00002B/399

9 781802 353969